ESSENTIAL TIPS

MASSAGE

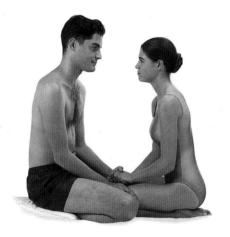

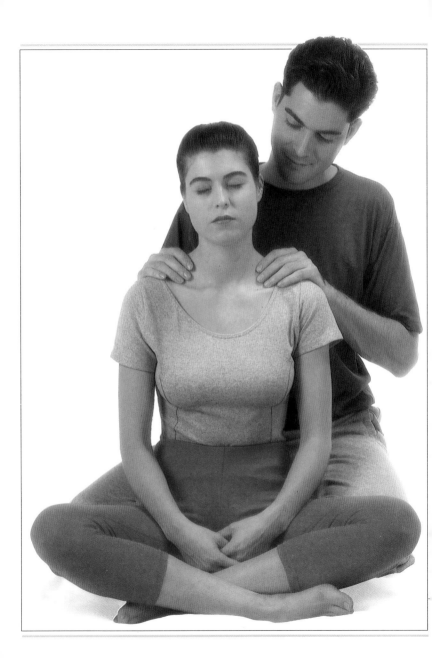

ESSENTIAL TIPS 101

MASSAGE

Nitya Lacroix

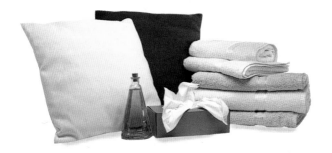

LONDON, NEW YORK, MELBOURNE,
MUNICH AND DELHI

Editor Charlotte Davies
Art Editor Ann Burnham
Managing Editor Gillian Roberts
Managing Art Editor Karen Sawyer
Category Publisher Mary-Clare Jerram
DTP Designer Sonia Charbonnier
Production Controller Luca Frassinetti

First published in Great Britain in 1995
This paperback edition published in Great Britain in 2003
by Dorling Kindersley Limited
80 Strand, London WC2R 0RL
Penguin Group (UK)

07 10 9 8 7 6 5 4

A CIP catalogue record for this book is available from The British Library

ISBN-13: 978-1-4053-0169-5
ISBN-10: 1-4053-0169-4

Colour reproduced by Colourscan, Singapore
Printed in China by WKT Company Limited

discover more at
www.dk.com

ESSENTIAL TIPS
101

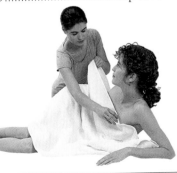

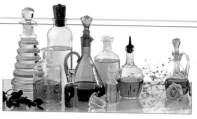

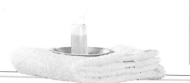

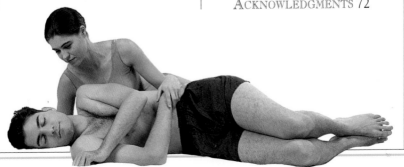

MASSAGE BENEFITS

1 WHAT IS MASSAGE?

Massage is an ancient form of healing, used for thousands of years to offer relief from pain, to restore good spirits, provide comfort, boost energy, and to rejuvenate muscles. It is a relaxing experience for giver and receiver. Massage uses touch to bring about emotional and physical changes, and to create a feeling of wholeness in the body and mind.

2 WHY USE MASSAGE?

The tactile action of massage has a great many useful effects. Massage will:
- Enhance one's awareness of body and breathing and so improve posture.
- Relieve accumulated tension and restore flexibility to tight, sore muscles.
- Break down waste products held in the muscles and improve the cleansing role of the lymphatic system.

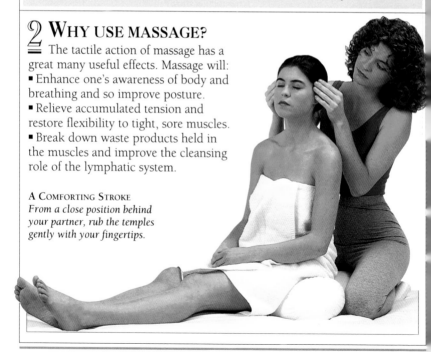

A COMFORTING STROKE
From a close position behind your partner, rub the temples gently with your fingertips.

3 SIGNS OF STRESS

The body is directly affected by the stress felt by everyone in their day-to-day lives – muscles tighten in response, and breath flow lessens.

These reactions are then reflected in a person's posture, which will alter according to where and how tension is held in various parts of the body.

The neck is bent, causing the head to be pushed forwards. It should be lengthened and brought in line with the spine

The jaw and face are tight with tension. They should be loose and supple

Tension in the shoulders has caused them to be rounded, instead of wide and relaxed

The chest is caved in and constricted. It needs to be opened out and widened

The spine is rigid and locked. It needs to be relaxed and extended upwards

Tension in the pelvis causes it to be locked back like this. It needs to drop forwards slightly, under the upper body

Instead of being loose and flexible, these legs are stiff with tension

The knees too are stiff and locked back. They should be loose and flexible

STRESS CONTROL
Some stress is inevitable in all our lives, but too much can lead to harmful emotional and physical side-effects. Learn to recognize the signs of tension in your body.

The upper body is leaning forwards. The feet should be stable and shoulder-width apart in order to support the body weight evenly

4 THE BODY'S RESPONSE TO MASSAGE

Massage actually speeds up the natural healing processes of the body, calms the mind, and settles the emotions. By reaching the emotions as well as the body, it evokes changes in the whole person. It is the perfect antidote to stress. To help your partner enjoy the benefits of massage, start by locating the points of tension around his body.

- Study his posture. Consider from top to toe where tension is held.
- Is his jaw tight? Circular strokes with the fingertips bring suppleness.
- Is his neck stiff? Soothing strokes will relieve sore shoulders, a stiff neck, and muscle contraction.
- Is his spine tense? Massaging the back will stretch and relieve rigid, tense muscles.

1 To relax the upper body, place your hands on the breastbone, fingers pointing inwards. Slide your hands around the shoulders and draw them up the back of the neck. Pull out through the hair.

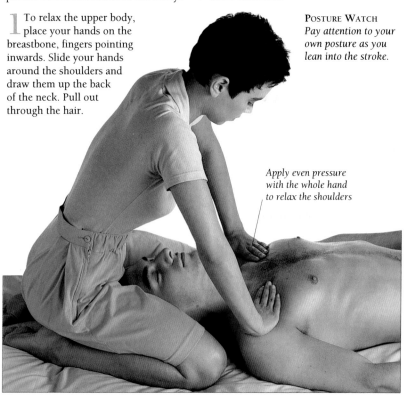

POSTURE WATCH
Pay attention to your own posture as you lean into the stroke.

Apply even pressure with the whole hand to relax the shoulders

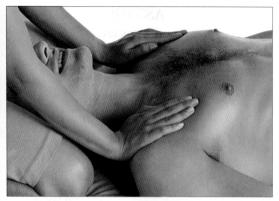

2 To relax the upper body further, place your hands flat on the shoulders with the heels of the hands on the shoulder muscle. Push downwards and outwards on the left shoulder. Gently release pressure, and repeat the same movement on the right shoulder. Build up to a rhythmic rocking action on both shoulders.

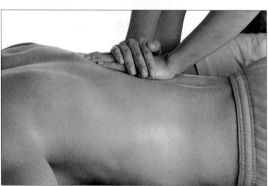

3 To ease back tension, relax the back with effleurage strokes (see p.26), then apply this spine stretch. Place your left hand on the lower back and add weight with your right hand. Use the flat of your hand with added pressure on the heel. Slide up the spine, and out through the arm. Repeat on other side.

5 WHEN NOT TO GIVE A MASSAGE

If your partner is suffering from any of the following, seek medical advice before going ahead with a massage, or indeed if you are in any doubt at all about appropriateness:
- High fever or skin condition.
- Swelling, undiagnosed lumps, inflammation, or heavy bruising.
- Recent scar tissue, fresh wounds, inflammation, or varicose veins.
- Acute back pain or severe injury.
- Cardiovascular conditions such as thrombosis or heart disease.
- Cancer, epilepsy, AIDS, or psychiatric illness of any kind.
- Pregnancy.

BEFORE YOU BEGIN

6 WHAT YOU NEED

Find a suitable surface on which to work, such as a futon, a foam rubber base, a thin mattress, or a massage table. Prepare an adequate supply of freshly washed sheets and towels. You will need a selection of large and small towels for use as coverings, plus some cushions. Keep carrier oil in a small bottle, or pour some into a saucer. Have tissues to hand to wipe away excess oil.

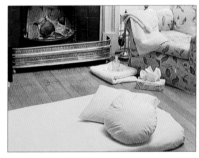

ORGANIZE THE ROOM IN ADVANCE
Keep everything you need close to hand.

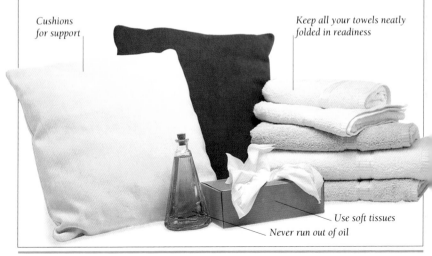

Cushions for support

Keep all your towels neatly folded in readiness

Use soft tissues

Never run out of oil

7 TIME IT RIGHT

A whole-body massage takes between an hour and an hour and a half, if you include the face and head. If your time is limited, concentrate on just one or two areas rather than rush through the whole body. A quick way to relax someone is to give a head and neck massage – this should last 15–20 minutes. A foot massage takes about 10 minutes per foot and is also deeply relaxing. A whole-back massage, the easiest kind for a beginner to give, should take 20 minutes.

MASSAGE FOR THE HEAD AND FACE
Spend 20 minutes on a head and face massage to calm and revitalize your partner and to soothe away tension trapped in the facial muscles.

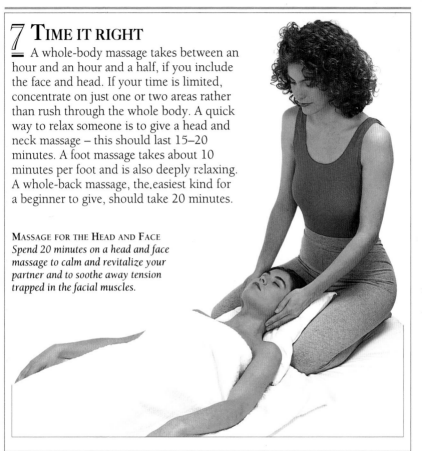

8 WHAT TO WEAR TO GIVE A MASSAGE

Ease of movement should be the main factor when choosing what to wear to give a massage – any comfortable, washable clothes will do. You need to be able to stretch with ease across the body and sit or kneel as the stroke requires.

- Wear comfortable, flat shoes or go barefoot – whichever you prefer.
- Remove any jewellery that may catch on the skin, and ask your massage partner to do the same.
- Keep your nails trimmed short. Long nails make strokes difficult.

9 SET THE SCENE

- Prepare the massage area to make it welcoming and comfortable.
- Remove clutter and make sure there is plenty of space to move freely around your massage partner.
- Ensure privacy and try to prevent any unnecessary interruptions.
- Avoid harsh, bright lighting.

10 EXTRA PADDING

Place cushions, pillows, or even rolled-up towels as props under your partner's body. This aids posture and helps relaxation, eases tension from various parts of the body, and loosens tight muscles. Put folded towels at the back of the head to take the strain off the neck.

11 CREATURE COMFORTS

Choose the most suitable surface on which to give your massage, such as a futon or a big piece of covered foam rubber. It should be large enough for your massage partner to lie on and for you to kneel on. Your partner must stay warm. Pre-heat the room and maintain the temperature. Open fires are particularly relaxing.

KEEP WARM
Maintain room temperature at 21° C (70° F).

If sitting alongside, support your pelvis with a cushion

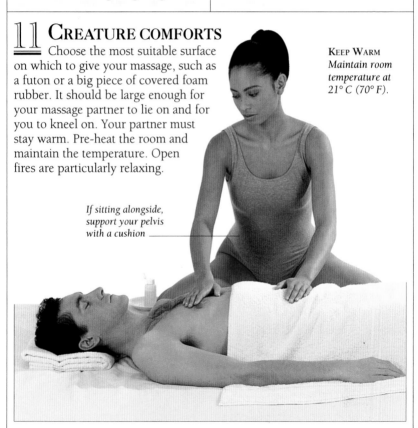

12 RELAX YOUR BREATHING

You must always breathe fully and evenly when giving a massage. Correct breathing calms the mind, unlocks energy, and frees tension. To achieve flowing breath, breathe deeply from the abdomen, allowing the breath to expand into the heart and chest area. Inhale through the nostrils and exhale through the mouth without forcing out.

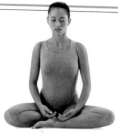

FOCUS ON YOUR BREATH

13 POSTURE CARE

Balanced posture is important when giving a massage. It gives you grace and helps you to breathe properly however you are giving the massage, so that you can finish feeling refreshed.

- Don't hunch your shoulders, or, in full-body massage, don't over-stretch.
- Keep your wrists loose and flexible.
- Lengthen the neck and spine.

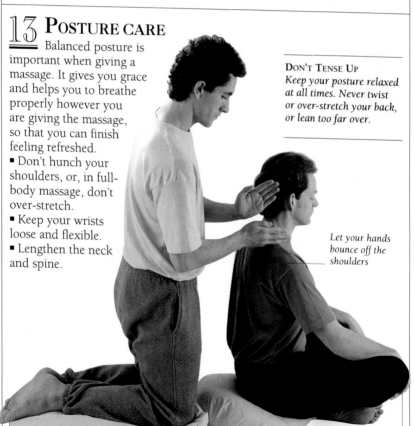

DON'T TENSE UP
Keep your posture relaxed at all times. Never twist or over-stretch your back, or lean too far over.

Let your hands bounce off the shoulders

14 TIME TO RELAX

Try to create an atmosphere of trust before you embark on your massage. This is most important if your partner has never had a massage before. He or she will feel tense and will not know what to expect. Do not rush straight in with your first stroke. Even before the initial touch, allow time for your partner's breathing to stabilize and for her to feel comfortably relaxed.

15 WHERE TO BEGIN

There is no right or wrong point at which to start. The back is one of the least threatening areas of the body and, as such, most people begin there, then complete with the front in order to put the recipient at ease. Others prefer to begin with a foot massage, which is equally relaxing. It is possible, however, to achieve a flowing, harmonious sequence from any starting point.

16 FOCUS ON HANDS

The quality of your touch is vital. To give an effective massage ideally your hands should be warm, attentive, dexterous, strong, and supple. Practise hand exercises to boost the confidence of your touch and to improve the range and creativity of your massage strokes.

- Concentrate on strengthening your hands, or your muscles will be tired and sore by the end of the massage.
- Study your hands to increase your awareness of them as creative tools.
- Use all parts of your hands.
- Don't forget that relaxed, supple hands are part of a relaxed body.

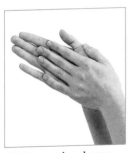

1 Vigorously rub your hands together to create heat and friction. Feel the heat and tingling sensation this generates.

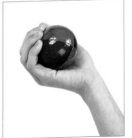

2 Clench and unclench on a soft juggling ball. This will increase the strength and suppleness of your palms and fingers.

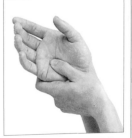

3 Ease tension out of the tendons and muscles by making circles with the thumb of one hand firmly into the palm of the other.

17 THE FIRST TOUCH

Only when you are sure that your partner is relaxed and comfortable should you make the initial contact. Approach the body slowly and sensitively. Begin the massage with an energy balancing hold of your choice (see p.21). A still hold over the spine is deeply relaxing. Let your hands rest there a while before continuing.

Touch the skin gently

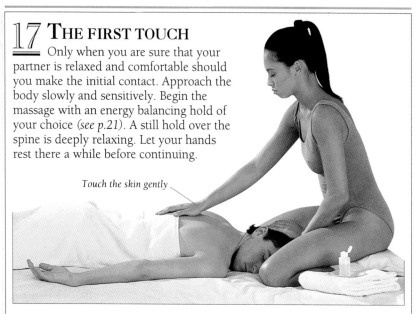

18 VARY THE PRESSURE

Different parts of the body require strokes of varying strengths. Increase the pressure by leaning your weight into the flat of your hand. Deepen the pressure further by placing the other hand on top. Apply deep, firm strokes to muscle-bound areas like the back but use gentle effleurage strokes to bony parts such as the ribcage.

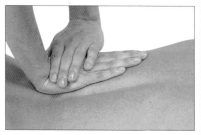

ADD YOUR WEIGHT TO THE STROKE

19 TICKLISHNESS

If your partner has a ticklish spot it is probably because he or she is nervous or tense. Take the stroke away from the ticklish area. Return to it later on in the massage when your partner is more relaxed.

20 HANDS ON

The quality of your touch will determine the quality of the massage you give. Your hands should display technical ability and dexterity, and should feel warm, and attentive. As you gain in experience, your touch will become more confident. Soon you will be able to sense the types of strokes your partner requires.

Observe the following to help you develop awareness of your hands and to realise their full potential.

- Study your hands. Appreciate that they are your creative tools.
- Exercise your hands regularly.
- Concentrate on your breathing as incorrect breathing will affect the quality of your touch.

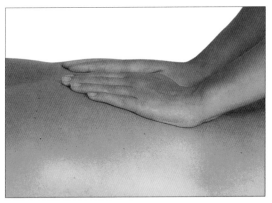

1 Use the flat of your hand to provide a relaxed, flowing effect. Place your hands on the body. Apply gentle, even pressure, keeping your wrists relaxed. Keep your thumbs and fingers in contact with the body so that the whole hands and not just the palms perform the stroke. This action relieves mental as well as physical tension.

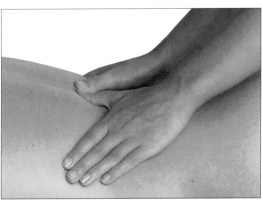

2 Use the tips of your thumbs to penetrate a specific area of tissue close to bones, such as along the spine. Place your whole hands on the body, with the fingers pointing away from the thumbs. Apply deep, even pressure with the tips of your thumbs. Keeping your thumbs dexterous will enable you to apply a wide range of strokes.

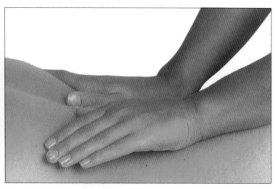

3 Apply deep pressure to tense muscles, leaning your weight into the inner edge of the heels and sides of the thumbs, while making circular movements with the hands, one hand following the other. Use this stroke to bring a feeling of relief to the lower back, the calves, and the soles of the feet.

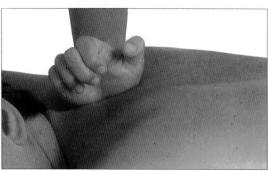

4 Rest the heel of your hand flat on your partner's body and apply even pressure. Keep the rest of your hand relaxed. The heel provides a broad, strong surface with which to ease away tension. Use to massage into tight muscle areas with circular motions, or to manipulate tissue.

21 FEEL THE RHYTHM

A good rhythm is essential for a successful massage. Any stroke feels good if it is applied in a flowing manner. Abrupt changes in tempo will disconcert your partner. Choose suitable music to set the pace of your massage, but keep the volume low. Don't allow the sound to be so loud that it intrudes and spoils the calming effects.

22 USE INTUITION

Massage is an intuitive form of therapy. You may feel uncertain about the sequence of strokes to follow but there is no rigid format to observe. You will become more confident as your experience grows. Your strokes will start to flow freely and you will be able to tell where and how deeply to apply them. Relax and trust your judgement.

23 CALMING TOUCHES

Don't be afraid to offer simple touches as well as specific massage strokes in your routine. Use the basic act of "laying on of hands" to create an awareness of breathing, and to bring about a feeling of stillness in you and your partner. Take the time to concentrate on the caring quality of your touch to enable you to reach and evoke changes in the mind and the body.

The simple touch of hands on the body instills a feeling of peace

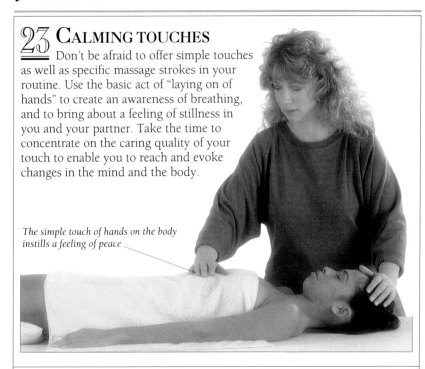

24 AVOID INTERRUPTIONS

Maintain hand-to-body contact with your partner as much as you can throughout the massage. If you lose your connection for a significant period you will interrupt the flow and disturb the recipient. During a sequence of strokes it is important that your partner experiences what feels like one flowing stroke. Keep oil refills and spare towels close to hand to minimize the impact if you need to pause for extra equipment.

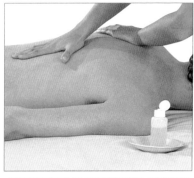

APPLY STROKES IN AN UNBROKEN SEQUENCE

25 CONNECTION HOLDS

Energy balancing or connection holds will bring a feeling of integration to your massage. Use them as a whole session in themselves, as a way to introduce and complete a massage, or as a method of connecting different parts of the body. They will help you and your partner to relax and give time for both of you to assimilate and enjoy the effects.

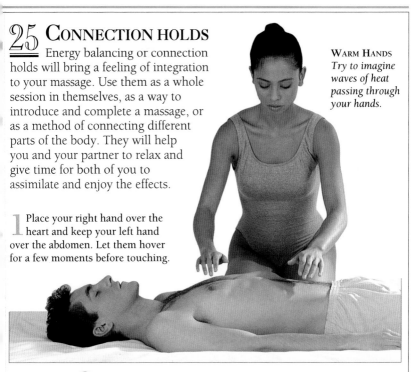

WARM HANDS
Try to imagine waves of heat passing through your hands.

1 Place your right hand over the heart and keep your left hand over the abdomen. Let them hover for a few moments before touching.

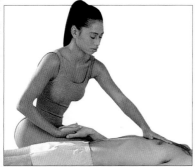

2 Rest one hand over the heart area to make contact with your partner's feelings and help with breathing.

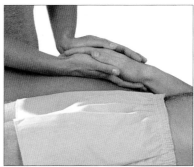

3 Take your partner's hand between your hands and hold it gently as a sign of warmth, affection, and trust.

21

26 POSTURAL EASE

Before you begin a massage, you should impart a sense of overall relaxation to your partner. Use these postural ease strokes to stretch and relax the principal areas of tension around your partner's body to give a sensation of length, width, and spaciousness. This will help your partner to lie down comfortably.

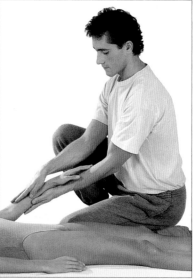

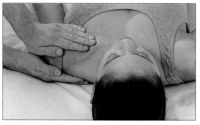

1 This sandwich hold will release the shoulder and bring width and space to the chest. Lift the shoulder and slip your right hand underneath. Point the fingers towards the spine. Enclose the area with the other hand. Pull out both hands firmly to the edge of the shoulder.

2 To give a feeling of length and release in the arms and shoulders, face your partner's arm and place your hands above and below the shoulder. Hold the arm firmly in both hands and pull into a downwards stretch. Draw the stroke out of your partner's fingertips.

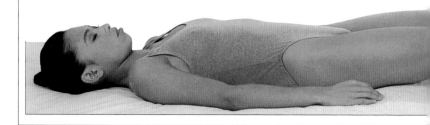

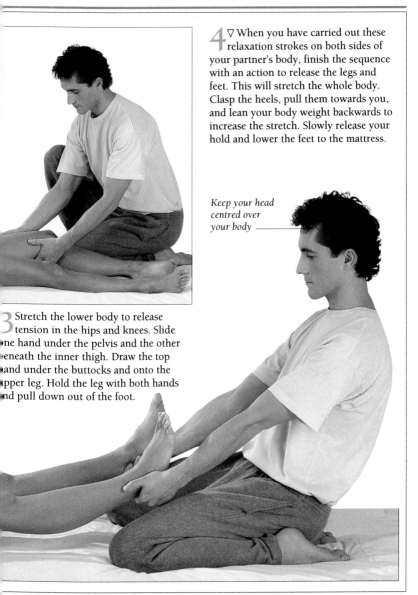

4 ▽ When you have carried out these relaxation strokes on both sides of your partner's body, finish the sequence with an action to release the legs and feet. This will stretch the whole body. Clasp the heels, pull them towards you, and lean your body weight backwards to increase the stretch. Slowly release your hold and lower the feet to the mattress.

Keep your head centred over your body ——

3 Stretch the lower body to release tension in the hips and knees. Slide one hand under the pelvis and the other beneath the inner thigh. Draw the top hand under the buttocks and onto the upper leg. Hold the leg with both hands and pull down out of the foot.

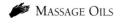
MASSAGE OILS

27 WHY USE OILS?

Oils are a necessary lubricant to prevent massage strokes from causing friction against the surface of the skin. They contain nutrients that are beneficial to the skin and tissue. Choose a carrier oil that is not sticky, and has no strong odour.

- Enrich your mix with luxurious peach, avocado, or almond oils.
- Use talcum powder instead of oil if necessary but always use oil for long, continuous strokes.
- Add drops of wheatgerm oil to the carrier to stop it from going rancid.

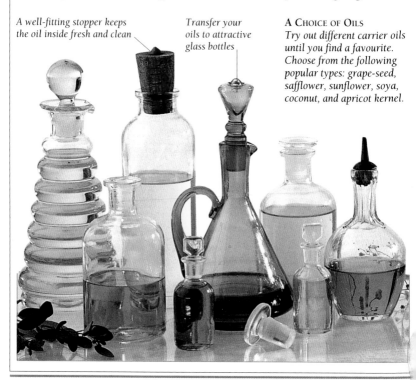

A well-fitting stopper keeps the oil inside fresh and clean

Transfer your oils to attractive glass bottles

A CHOICE OF OILS
Try out different carrier oils until you find a favourite. Choose from the following popular types: grape-seed, safflower, sunflower, soya, coconut, and apricot kernel.

28 HOW MUCH OIL?

For initial application, pour about one teaspoon of oil onto your hands for spreading on the body. You will need about 30 ml (1 fl oz) for a whole-body massage. There should be enough oil on the skin to ensure a smooth stroke.

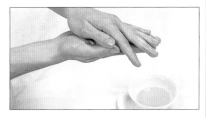

TOO MUCH OIL WILL MAKE THE SKIN STICKY

29 HOW TO SPREAD OIL

Squeeze or drip the oil into the palm of one hand. Be careful not to drip oil onto your partner's body. Rub the oil into your hands to warm them and spread the oil over the body with smooth, flowing strokes. Do not use too much oil to begin with. It is better to add more if you need it rather than to have to wipe away excess from the skin surface.

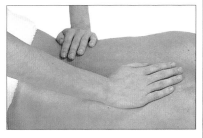

SPREAD THE OIL EVENLY OVER THE BACK

30 KEEP COVERED

An oiled body loses heat quickly, so always put towels over exposed areas. Do not let the relaxing effects of your massage go to waste by letting the body temperature drop.

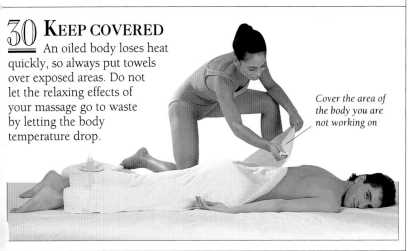

Cover the area of the body you are not working on

THE BACK & SHOULDERS

31 EFFLEURAGE ON THE BACK

Relax the back with a sequence of smooth, flowing effleurage strokes, the principal strokes of massage. Use them on the back to stretch the muscles and to boost the cardiovascular system. Rest both hands on either sides of the spine, then slide them down the long muscles of the back, as far as you can reach comfortably. Fan your hands out to the sides of the body. Mould them around the contours of the ribcage, and draw them around the shoulder blades and out towards the shoulders in one continuous movement.

ALL-OVER ADVANTAGES
The continuous, rounded movements are psychologically and physically soothing; they benefit the nervous system and reduce stress.

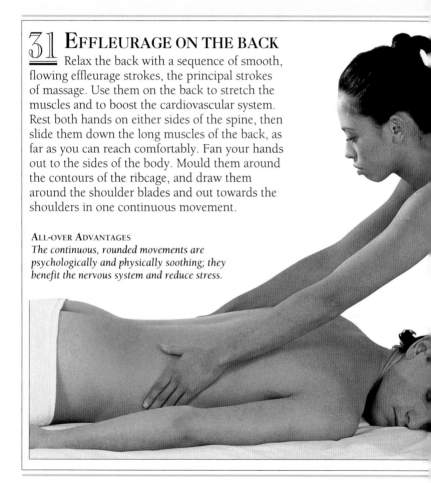

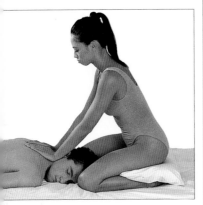

SMOOTH SEQUENCE
Apply effleurage to the back using the flat of the hand at a constant pressure. Use before and after deeper strokes to prepare the body beforehand and to soothe it afterwards.

32 EASE TENSION

To complete this effleurage stroke on the back, continue by pulling your hands across the tops of the shoulders to the base of the neck. Don't drag on the shoulders. When your hands reach the neck, sweep them up and over the neck and right out through the head. Repeat the stroke several times.

NECK RELEASE
This satisfying stroke relaxes muscles in the back and neck.

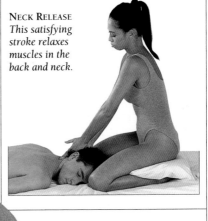

APPLYING EFFLEURAGE
Effleurage can be used all over the body, not just on the back, to prepare the area for subsequent techniques. Never end effleurage strokes abruptly. Round them off gradually or draw them out of the body. Ask your partner to advise you on the pressure of the strokes.

33 FAN STROKES

Use this effleurage stroke to relax and lengthen muscles after the main strokes and before deeper work. Place your hands flat on the back at the base of the spine. Glide them gently up the back and then fan them out to mould the sides of the body, and pull down. Turn your wrists out and glide your hands back to the source of the stroke. Let each stroke flow into the next.

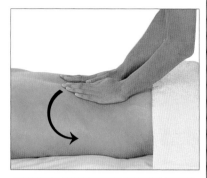

LEAN YOUR BODY WEIGHT INTO THE STROKE

34 CIRCULAR STROKES

The trick of this more complex stroke is to achieve an unbroken circular motion. Place both hands parallel on the lower side of the body and start to slide them in a circular motion. Then lift your right hand off the body to allow the left hand underneath to finish its full circle, before dropping the right hand back down. Cover the surface of the back. Use circular strokes to loosen and relax muscles on the back, belly, and the sides of the ribcage.

Pass the right hand over the left hand

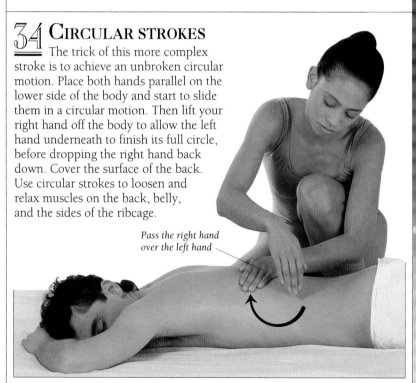

35 SIDE STROKES

Use side strokes (or cross-over strokes as they are also known) to work the superficial tissue of the muscles. Take the strokes along from the lower back, up to the shoulder blades, and back down again. This will lengthen the back muscles and create gentle friction on the base and middle of the back.

- Do not interrupt the stroke – it should be continuous and flowing.
- Focus on the areas of the lower back that are tense and contracted.
- Keep your own posture in mind, particularly when leaning across to reach your partner's far side.
- Change the pace of your strokes. Start slowly, then increase speed.

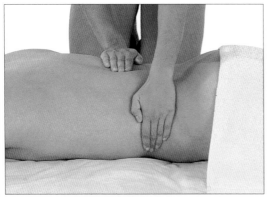

1 Begin by positioning yourself comfortably by your partner's side. Mould your hands, with your fingers pointing away from you, over both sides of the back. Let your fingertips slip just under the front of your partner's body on the opposite side. Apply firm but gentle pressure with the palm of the hand and the length of the fingers.

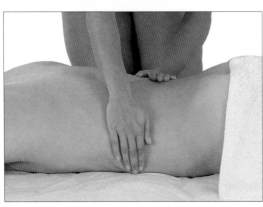

2 Slide your hands past each other to opposite sides of the back. Glide the heel of your hand firmly down the side nearest to you to meet the edge of the mattress. Repeat this movement continuously, swapping hands from one side to the other. Move your hands up and down your partner's body as you go, a little at a time.

36 STRETCH THE BACK

Stretches are firm, sliding movements that promote a feeling of length and breadth in the body. Give them to relieve tension in the back. They can also be used on the sides of the body, and the arms and legs. Spine stretches feel good since they bring a feeling of relief.

1 ▷ Place the flats of your hands side by side in the centre of the back. For maximum effect, slide them in opposite directions using slow, steady pressure.

2 Glide your right hand from the centre of the back to the base of the neck. Draw your left hand down the lower back to the sacrum. Let your hands rest in an energy balancing hold.

Do not press on the vertebrae when applying a stretch

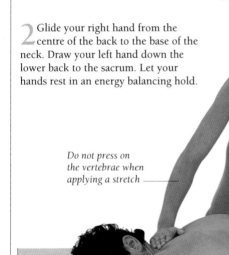

37 HOW TO FEATHER

Trace the tips of your fingers lightly down the surface of the back in a flowing unbroken movement. Use this delicate action to create a tingling sensation, or apply feather strokes to end a massage following effleurage strokes.

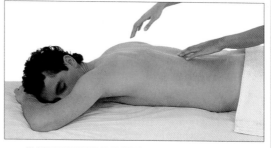

IF YOUR PARTNER IS TICKLISH INCREASE THE PRESSURE

38 KNEAD THE BACK

Kneading is the second stage of massage. Apply it only when the muscles have been warmed up with soothing strokes. Lift and squeeze a portion of flesh in one hand and roll it towards the other hand. Repeat the action back and forth. Knead the flesh on the buttocks, along the side of the body, and over the outer edges of the shoulder blades. Then knead thoroughly over the shoulders to the base of the neck.

LOOSEN UP
Knead to relax the network of muscles in the upper back.

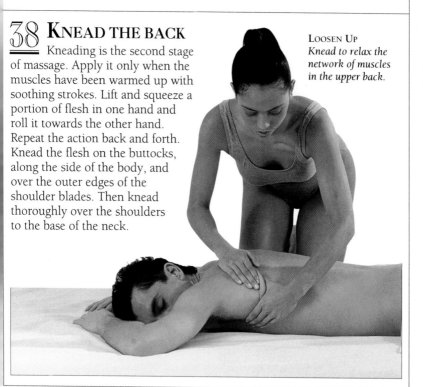

31

39 KNEAD A TIGHT SPOT

Apply firm kneading strokes along the top of the shoulders. Focus the action on the narrow area of flesh in between the top edge of the shoulder blades and the base of the neck. Roll the muscles from one hand to the other to release pent-up tension carried in the neck. Without relief, this tension can lead to stiffnes.

ALL-OVER BENEFITS
Relaxed shoulders will reduce mental anxiety.

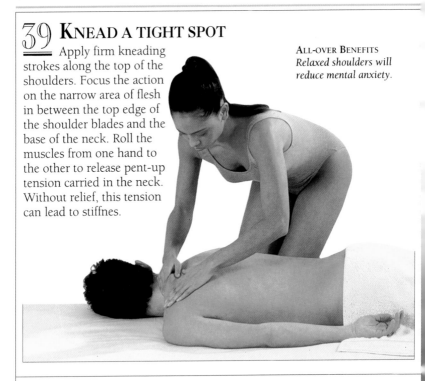

40 KNEAD BOTH SHOULDERS

Hook your fingers over your partner's shoulders, scoop the flesh with your heels and thumbs, then alternately squeeze and release the flesh. Continue kneading well.

- Warm the muscles with soothing strokes before you begin to knead.
- Manipulate the flesh until you feel stiff shoulder muscles loosen.
- Follow up with effleurage.

41 PETRISSAGE ON THE BACK

Petrissage is a deep massage stroke used for pushing areas of tissue towards the bone. Prepare the back with effleurage and kneading.

- Sink your fingertips, thumbs, or heels into tissue and make small circles or firm short slides.
- Apply pressure sensitively.

42 WORK THE SPINE

Apply petrissage strokes to relax the spine and bring relief to the whole body. Petrissage on the back corrects the posture by easing tension from the length of the spine, bringing relief to stiff ligaments, and increasing flexibility in the muscles that support the spine. These deep, penetrating strokes will also serve to disperse toxins and trapped waste products into the circulatory system for elimination from the body.

TROUBLE SPOTS
Manipulate areas of knotted tension.

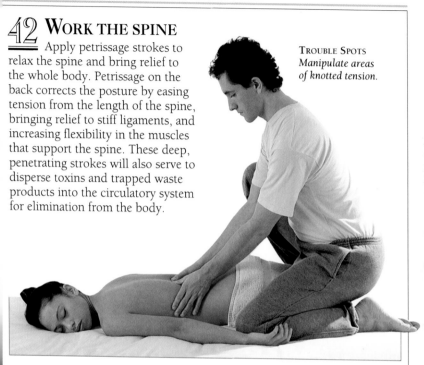

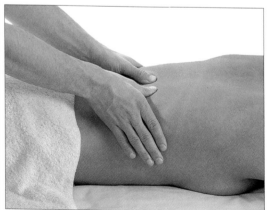

1 △ Facing the direction of the stroke, press your thumb pads firmly into the grooves on either side of the vertebrae, while resting your hands at an angle.

2 ◁ Work your thumbs up from the base of the spine in a single long, smooth movement. At the shoulder blades, glide your hands up over the shoulders and down the sides of the body.

33

43 WORK THE SACRUM

The sacrum is a flat bone at the base of the spine which also forms part of the pelvic girdle. Day-to-day poor posture and muscular strain create a build-up of tension in the sacrum and lower back. Massage to this area feels deeply satisfying.

- Relax the sacrum before and after petrissage with soothing strokes.
- Do not apply too much massage oil as this will prevent your fingers from penetrating the muscles.
- Massage around this area to give comfort and to relieve stress.

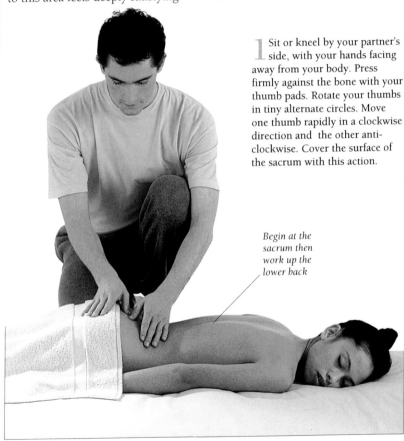

1 Sit or kneel by your partner's side, with your hands facing away from your body. Press firmly against the bone with your thumb pads. Rotate your thumbs in tiny alternate circles. Move one thumb rapidly in a clockwise direction and the other anti-clockwise. Cover the surface of the sacrum with this action.

Begin at the sacrum then work up the lower back

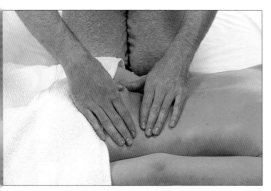

2 Place your right hand above the sacrum with your thumb at an angle, pointing away from your fingers. Push it firmly towards your left hand to create a degree of slack in the muscles surrounding the sacrum. Carry on making small, grinding circles against the bone using the thumb pad of your right hand.

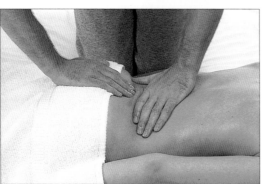

3 Raise your kneeling position to give greater weight to your hands. Use your left hand to push up against the sacrum. Swivel your right wrist so that your fingertips point up the back. Cup your hand over the buttocks and apply steady pressure on the sacrum with your fingertips. Make small circles over the bone.

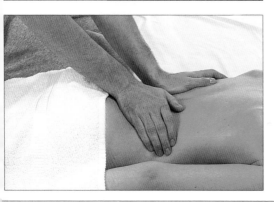

4 Move to kneel facing the head in order to continue the massage further up the back. Apply pressure with the sides and heels of the thumbs to make alternate fan strokes. Start off at the sacrum and move up the back. Apply pressure in an upward and outward continous motion, one hand following the other.

44 RELAXING THE SPINE

Place your hands at a slight angle on both sides of the spine and apply pressure with the thumbs. Slide your thumbs down the back as far as you can reach. Sweep your hands up around the sides of the body and over the shoulders. Repeat the stroke at least twice.

- Use to relieve tight ligaments, to release tension, and to bring extra flexibility to the supporting muscles.
- Apply only after effleurage strokes.
- Never push on a muscle area too quickly or the body will contract.
- Increase the pressure gradually with each repetition of the stroke.

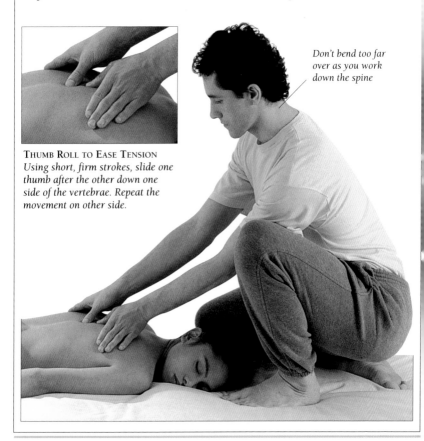

Don't bend too far over as you work down the spine

THUMB ROLL TO EASE TENSION
Using short, firm strokes, slide one thumb after the other one side of the vertebrae. Repeat the movement on other side.

45 SPINAL HOLD

On a physical level, an energy balancing hold links different parts of the body, and on an emotional level, it encourages a feeling of integration. A connection hold to the back serves both purposes by promoting a sense of unity from the top to the base of the back, and by releasing tension held in the spine.

THE SIMPLE TOUCH
Using the minimum of touch, this basic spinal hold brings about deep-seated benefits to both mind and body.

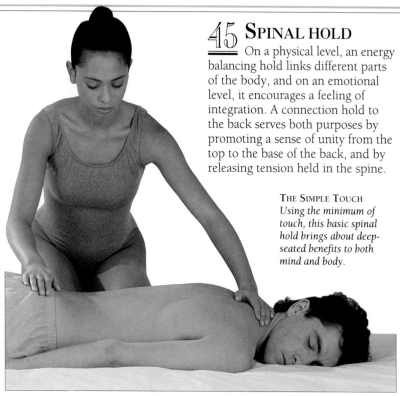

1 △ Place one hand on the top of the neck so that it rests on the vertebrae responsible for movement of the head. This will feel deeply comforting for the recipient. Create a feeling of balance in the spine by gently laying the other hand at the base of the back, over the sacrum.

2 ▷ Hold your hands just above the centre of the spine and slowly and gently lower them onto the vertebrae. Try to imagine your breath flowing like an energizing electric current from your hands to your partner's body.

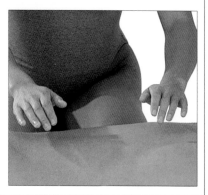

MASSAGE FOR THE LOWER BODY

46 STROKE THE LEGS

There are many extra benefits to a soothing leg massage. It can lift strain and tension from the lower body, and this brings relief to a tight, sore back. The main stroke warms, soothes, and stretches the whole leg and will invigorate a sluggish circulation with its upward action. Begin by applying oil with downward strokes to the whole leg.

1 Place your hands parallel over the back of the ankles. Glide the hands smoothly up over the contours of the calf.

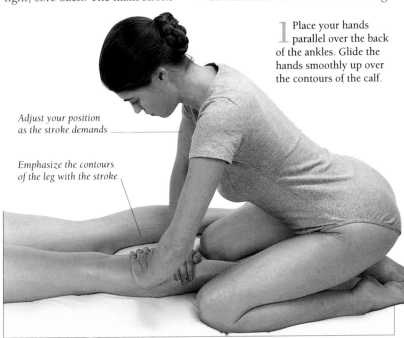

Adjust your position as the stroke demands

Emphasize the contours of the leg with the stroke

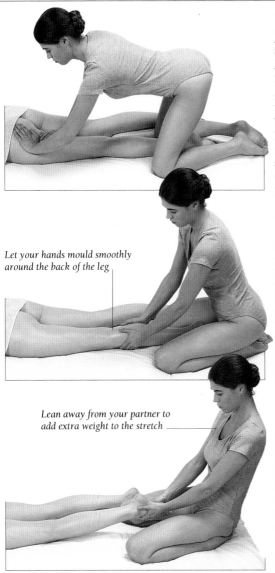

Let your hands mould smoothly around the back of the leg

Lean away from your partner to add extra weight to the stretch

2 Lean your weight into the stroke as you slide your hands up the leg. Lessen the pressure from your hands as you pass the back of the knee. Lean forwards to slip your leading hand around the buttocks and the other hand to wait on the inner thigh. Your moving hand should then slide down over the hip to the outer part of the thigh.

3 When both hands are placed equally on the thigh, slide your fingers under either side of the leg. Support the leg with your hands and pull firmly down from the thigh to the ankle. Lean back into a more upright position as you approach the ankle to create a gentle but firm stretch in the hip and groin region.

4 When you reach the ankle, slide one hand under the upper foot and the other over the sole. Lean right back on your heels, pull gently on the leg, and take the stroke out of the ends of the toes. Repeat all strokes on the other leg. This is a satisfying conclusion to the massage session for the lower body.

39

47 KNEAD THE CALVES

Sit at your partner's feet. Place the heels of your hands and thumbs in the centre of the calf, with the fingers wrapped lightly round the front of the leg. Move your hands up the leg, one after the other, in a continuous, circular action. Work your hands up to the back of the knee and glide down.

- Precede and follow up kneading strokes with main strokes to warm up and relax the calf muscles.
- Squeeze the flesh with each outward movement of the circle.
- Apply pressure gently as the calves are highly sensitive.
- Repeat the entire sequence of strokes on the other calf.

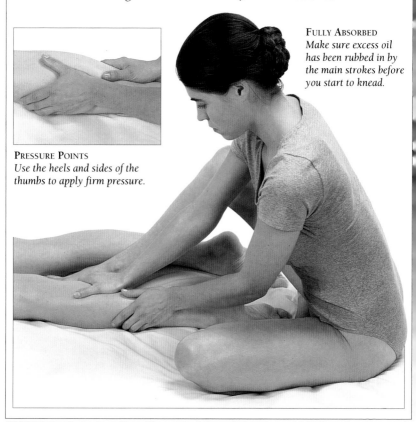

FULLY ABSORBED
Make sure excess oil has been rubbed in by the main strokes before you start to knead.

PRESSURE POINTS
Use the heels and sides of the thumbs to apply firm pressure.

48 KNEAD THE LEGS AND BUTTOCKS

Place both hands on your partner's thigh with your fingers facing away and the thumbs at an angle. Anchor the hold with your thumbs and scoop the flesh with one hand, squeeze it between the thumb and forefingers, and roll it to the other hand. Create a wave of flesh moving between both hands.

- First apply effleurage strokes.
- Use kneading strokes on both legs to boost the blood supply and to increase the exchange of tissue fluid.
- Incorporate the buttocks in a massage to the back or to the legs.
- Use kneading on the buttocks to relieve emotional, physical, or sexual tension held in the muscles.

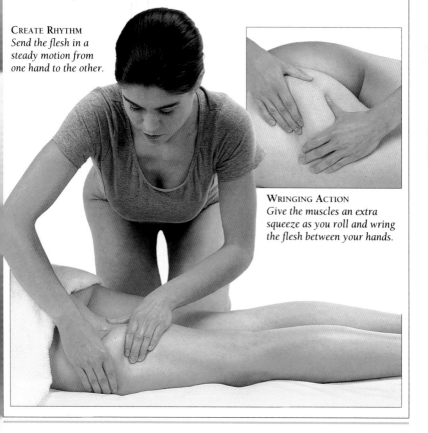

CREATE RHYTHM
Send the flesh in a steady motion from one hand to the other.

WRINGING ACTION
Give the muscles an extra squeeze as you roll and wring the flesh between your hands.

49 FINISH OFF

Follow up kneading strokes with effleurage and then conclude the massage to the lower body with invigorating percussion strokes. From a position beside your partner, strike the buttocks and the backs of the legs with the sides of your hands. Try to maintain a rhythmic, brisk action, keeping your hands, arms, and shoulders as relaxed as possible. If your hands become tense then the strokes will feel like karate chops. The rapid action of the hands bouncing against the body improves muscle tone, stimulates the nerve endings, and draws the blood supply up to the skin.

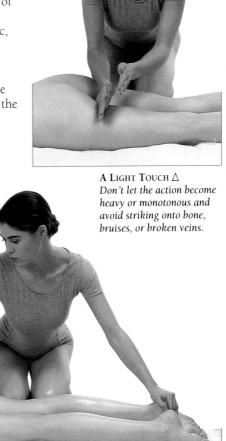

A LIGHT TOUCH △
Don't let the action become heavy or monotonous and avoid striking onto bone, bruises, or broken veins.

CONNECTION HOLD ▽
After giving percussion strokes, link both halves of the body by placing one hand on the soles of the feet and the other on the sacrum. Hold your hands in position for one minute.

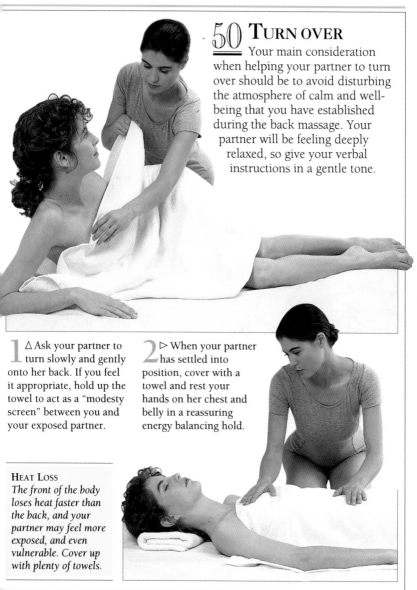

50 TURN OVER

Your main consideration when helping your partner to turn over should be to avoid disturbing the atmosphere of calm and well-being that you have established during the back massage. Your partner will be feeling deeply relaxed, so give your verbal instructions in a gentle tone.

1 △ Ask your partner to turn slowly and gently onto her back. If you feel it appropriate, hold up the towel to act as a "modesty screen" between you and your exposed partner.

2 ▷ When your partner has settled into position, cover with a towel and rest your hands on her chest and belly in a reassuring energy balancing hold.

HEAT LOSS
The front of the body loses heat faster than the back, and your partner may feel more exposed, and even vulnerable. Cover up with plenty of towels.

THE HEAD & FACE

51 TAKE CONTROL

Stress and anxiety are key factors in the build-up of tension and the head, face, and neck are prone to tension stiffness. This can be effectively relieved by massage, but your partner must relax, let go of everyday habits, and allow you to take full charge. Be confident with your hands so that you can freely manipulate the head and neck.

52 HOW TO SIT

For upper body work, place yourself behind your partner's head. Use a cushion to support your pelvis and tilt it forwards. Do not begin your sequence of strokes until you feel completely comfortable. Keep your spine lengthened and try to avoid hunching your shoulders.

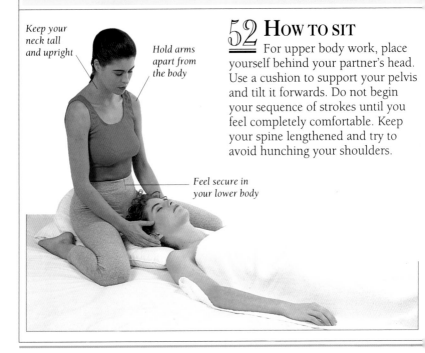

Keep your neck tall and upright

Hold arms apart from the body

Feel secure in your lower body

Assist breathing and keep your body relaxed by holding your chest and shoulders wide open

53 NECK EXTENSION

Use this stroke to bring alignment to the neck, to relieve tension caused by contracted muscles, and to help the neck to extend away from the shoulders. Allow sufficient time for your partner's neck to relax into your hands before you begin the stroke.

1 Scoop your hands underneath your partner's shoulders and rest them, with the palms facing upwards, on either side of the spinal column.

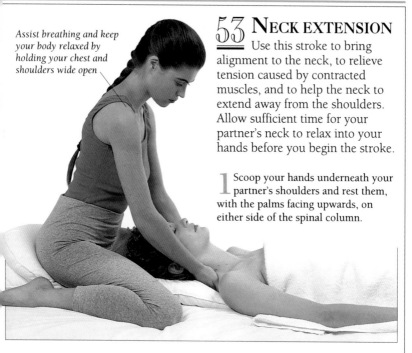

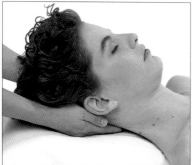

2 As the neck relaxes, glide your hands towards you, ensuring that the neck is fully supported by them. Lift the head as your hands pass under the hairline.

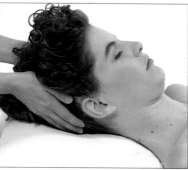

3 Draw your hands steadily under and out of the head, extending the stroke away from the body. Repeat until the neck feels completely loose and relaxed.

54 CROWN HOLDS

These still, relaxing holds will soothe an overactive mind, relieve stress, and alleviate physical tension. Use them to bring calmness and integration to a massage. They can be given at the beginning or the end of a whole-body massage, or used to start off a massage to the head and face, or neck and shoulders.

- Focus attention on your breath. Imagine it sending warmth and vitality to your hands and fingers.
- Keep your eyes closed to help focus and maintain concentration.
- Spend about 30 seconds per hold, longer if your partner seems restless.
- Try to convey a feeling of calm and attentiveness with your hands.

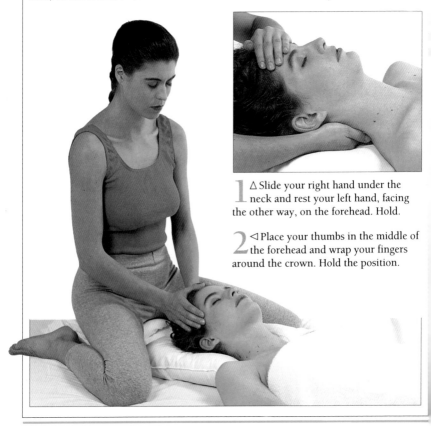

1 △ Slide your right hand under the neck and rest your left hand, facing the other way, on the forehead. Hold.

2 ◁ Place your thumbs in the middle of the forehead and wrap your fingers around the crown. Hold the position.

55 RELEASE THE HEAD

Induce a feeling of relaxation, security, and relief by supporting the weight of your partner's head in your hands and lifting and rolling it. Pause at any point if you can feel resistance against the movement of your hands. Find the pivotal point at the top of the spine from which to turn the head from side to side.

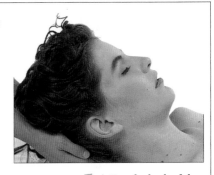

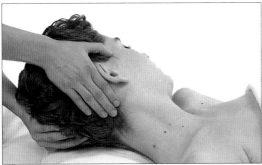

1 △ Cup the back of the head and, keeping it in line with the spine, lift it up and stretch the neck. Lower it to let the weight drop gently in your hands.

2 ◁ Lift the head and turn it to rest in your left palm while supporting it with your other hand. Then roll it to lie facing in the opposite direction.

56 STROKE THE BROWS

Use this soothing stroke to relax the forehead. Place your thumbs just above the brow bone. Apply gentle pressure with the thumb pads. Glide your thumbs steadily outwards from the centre to the outer sides of the brow and complete the stroke with a sweep of the temples. Move your thumbs up a little to stroke in a similar way over the whole area. Withdraw your thumbs smoothly and gently from contact with the face.

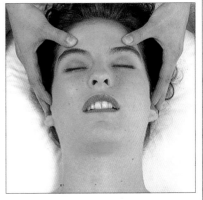

USE THUMB PADS FIRMLY BUT GENTLY

57 STROKE THE EYES

Give an eye massage to ease tension and headaches, to help clear sinus passages, and as an effective way to relieve stress and lift away tiredness from the eyes and body.

- Never press on the sensitive eye socket area or drag the delicate skin.
- Contact lenses should be removed before massaging the eye area.
- Use a confident, sensitive touch.

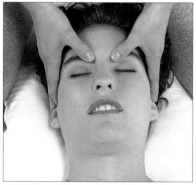

1 Enclose the temples with your fingers and press the thumb pads into the pressure points at the edge of the brows.

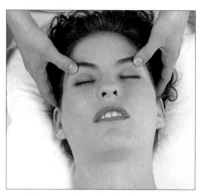

2 Slide your thumb pads firmly along the eyebrows as far as their outer corners. Keep your pressure steady.

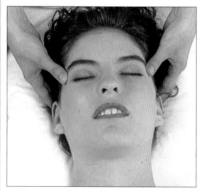

3 Press gently into the last pressure point on the outer edge of the brow. Follow with a sweep around the temples.

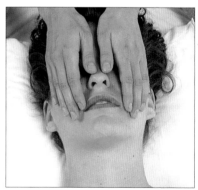

4 Rest your palms over the eye sockets without applying pressure. Allow the eyes to feel the warmth of your hands.

58 LOOSEN THE CHEEKS

People often disguise their feelings by unconsciously tightening their facial muscles, particularly around the cheeks and mouth. This muscular tension leads to a visible mask-like effect. Apply circular petrissage strokes with the tips of your fingers over the cheek area to loosen the muscles and to alleviate the discomfort of facial tension.

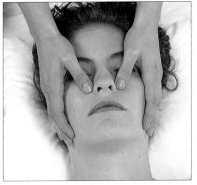

1 Glide your thumb pads down from the bridge of the nose and slide them into the muscle below the cheekbone.

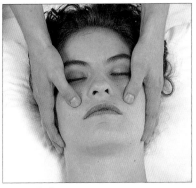

2 Apply firm, even pressure as you draw your thumbs underneath the cheekbones and out towards the ears.

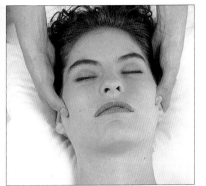

3 Take the stroke to the sides of the head and sweep your hands out over the scalp to the ends of the hair.

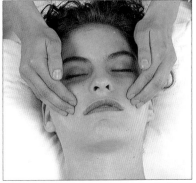

4 Press your fingertips into the fleshy areas of the cheeks and make several small circles, one area at a time.

59 KNEAD THE JAW

The jaw muscles are among the strongest muscles in the whole body. However, as with all parts of the face, you must still use a steady but sensitive touch. Apply circular, kneading strokes outwards from the chin along each side of the jaw.

60 STROKE THE JAW

After kneading, apply gentle, soothing strokes that follow the contours of the jawline. The action of these strokes, combined with the warm and comforting touch of your hands, will cause your partner's face to soften and relax noticeably.

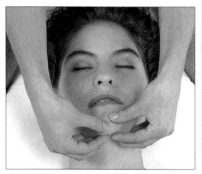

1 Grip the chin with your thumbs and forefingers. Make small, circular strokes, one thumb following the other.

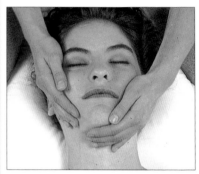

1 Very lightly stroke the throat with your fingertips. Then use the flat of your hands to stroke the jaw and chin.

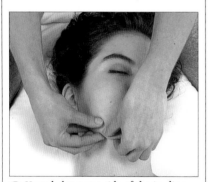

2 Knead along one side of the jawline, with sliding strokes, moving up towards the ear. Repeat on the other side.

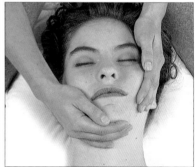

2 Use alternate hands to make outward, sweeping strokes under both sides of the jaw. Apply firm but gentle pressure.

61 RUB THE EARS

A massage on and around the ears has a surprisingly relaxing effect on the whole body. Take hold of each ear between your thumbs and your fingertips. Make tiny circles, squeezing gently as you go. Work on both ears simultaneously.

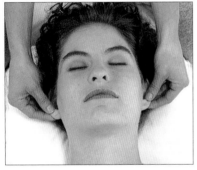

1 Work carefully over the ear lobes in a continuous, circular action. Press the thumbs gently over the rim of the ears.

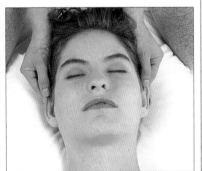

2 Lightly stroke inside the folds of both ears, and the area surrounding, with the tips of your middle and index fingers.

62 SCALP MASSAGE

Make brisk petrissage strokes with your fingertips from the base of the neck to the crown to loosen the thin layer of muscle over the skull.

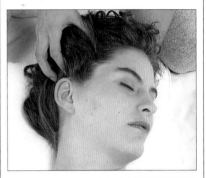

RUB THE SCALP AS IF SHAMPOOING THE HAIR

63 DRAW HANDS OUT

Bring a face, head, and scalp massage to a relaxing and hypnotic conclusion by combing your fingers through to the ends of the hair.

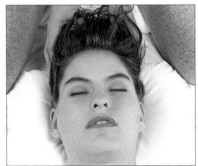

RELEASE THE LAST TRACES OF TENSION

MASSAGE FOR THE NECK & CHEST

64 RELAX THE NECK

To ease taut neck muscles, place one hand beneath the base of the neck and squeeze the flesh. Pull your hand towards you, and as it leaves the body, bring in your other hand so that the stroking motion is continuous, like pulling on a rope. This milking action increases the circulation of blood to the brain, thus relieving tension headaches.

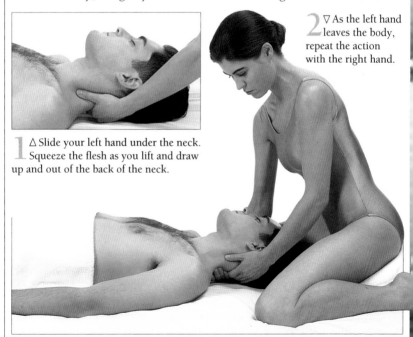

△ Slide your left hand under the neck. Squeeze the flesh as you lift and draw up and out of the back of the neck.

2 ▽ As the left hand leaves the body, repeat the action with the right hand.

65 CONNECT WITH THE CHEST

Before moving onto chest strokes, make a link between the head and chest. This will draw your partner's attention to the heart area. With your fingers straight, place the palm of your left hand against the temple, your thumb resting on the forehead. Rest your right hand on the chest. Hold for a few moments.

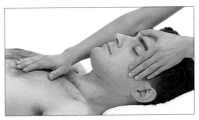

THIS HOLD HAS A SEDATIVE EFFECT

66 WORK THE RIBCAGE

The chest harbours vulnerable feelings and a massage here will make contact with these emotions. These strokes ease tension by relieving muscular constriction. As the muscles relax, so breathing becomes deeper. Repeat each sequence three times.

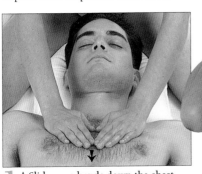

1 △ Slide your hands down the chest, fan out to the ribs, up to the armpits and back to the chest. Repeat twice more.

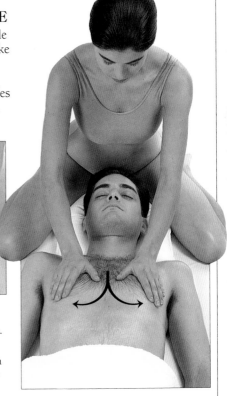

2 ▷ Relax the chest with shorter fan strokes. Glide both hands down then outwards. Draw your hands up the sides of the ribcage and into the next stroke.

67 PRESS ON THE SHOULDERS

Loosen up and expand the upper chest by pushing your own weight down through your hands onto both shoulders. Place a cupped hand on each shoulder and apply a steady, downward pressure. The chest will open and rise up, while the shoulders will drop down to the mattress. Hold for a few seconds, then release the pressure slowly.

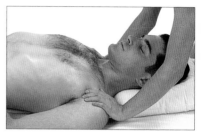

RELAX HUNCHED OR STIFF SHOULDERS

68 PECTORAL MASSAGE

Pectoral muscles are responsible for the movement of the shoulder blades and arms. The release of physical tension from the pectorals through massage brings a feeling of width to the shoulders. Be aware however that physical tension held in this part of the body could be rooted in emotional stress, and its release may cause the release of suppressed feelings.

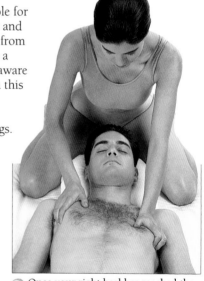

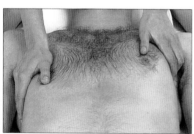

1 Hook the fingertips of both hands round the pectorals and push the heel of your right hand firmly from the collar bone out to the armpit. Lean your weight steadily into the stroke. Keep your left hand anchored in place on the other side.

2 Once your right heel has reached the armpit, lift it off the body and push down with the left hand. Don't let both hands leave the body at the same time. This stroke is known as the "cat paw" due to its rhythmic, pawing action.

69 HEART TO ABDOMINAL HOLD

Make a connection between the chest and abdomen before moving on to the abdominal area. Kneel at your partner's side and lay one hand over the heart and the other over the belly. This will create a feeling of harmony between the upper and lower halves of the torso. Hold the position to encourage connection and deeper breathing.

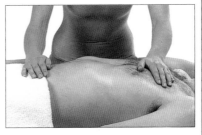

HANDS SHOULD FEEL SOFT AND WARM

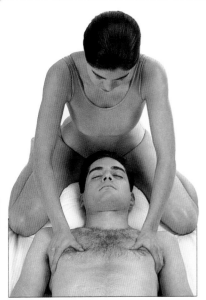

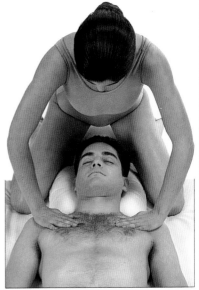

3 Anchor your fingertips around the armpits and knead the muscles above the breast area by making simultaneous circular strokes with the heels of both hands. Apply greater pressure on the outward slide and less on the return.

4 Finish off the pectoral massage with spreading strokes. Place your hands together on the breastbone. Draw them up towards you and then out towards the shoulders. If necessary, use extra oil to avoid painful dragging on chest hair.

THE BELLY

70 APPROACH WITH CAUTION

Like the chest, the belly not only contains vital organs, but also holds powerful emotions. Because of this many people find it hard to allow this area to be touched.

- Approach slowly and carefully.
- Make your opening contact a gentle touch just under the ribcage.
- Treat all parts of the body with respect, but especially the abdomen.

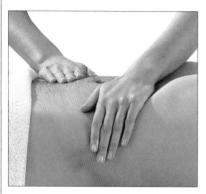

71 CIRCULAR STROKES

Open your massage with a connection hold from the upper to the lower abdomen. When you are sure that your partner is relaxed, proceed with your strokes. Circular strokes are the basic effleurage strokes for the abdomen. Use them to connect with the emotionally vulnerable side of your partner, to ease nervous tension held in the abdomen, and to assist digestion.

1 △ Start by slowly sliding the palms of both hands in large, circular strokes in a clockwise motion. Make the circles smaller and smaller to focus on the centre of the belly. Then expand them again to the outer edges of the abdomen.

2 ▷ Raise the right hand to allow the other hand to make a full circle. Return the raised hand to the body to trace the crescent shape of the last half of the circle. These strokes create a hypnotic effect and as your partner relaxes you can increase the pressure.

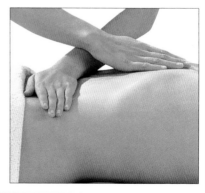

72 FIGURE-OF-EIGHT

Use this stroke to relax the sides of the body and the lower back as well as the sensitive belly area. In order to achieve a flowing figure-of-eight shape you will need to be able to move one hand clockwise and the other anti-clockwise simultaneously. This action requires practice to perfect good coordination between the left and right hand. Don't worry if, to begin with, you have difficulty making the figure-of-eight shape. It will come with time.

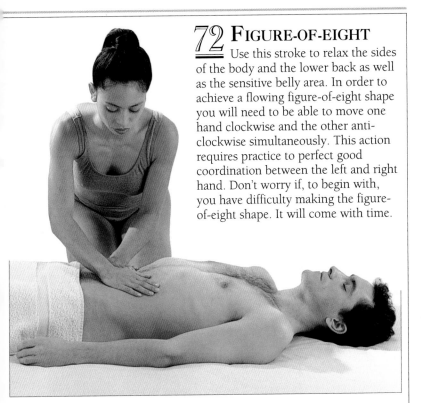

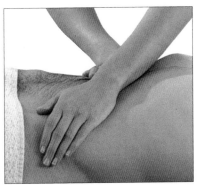

1 △ Kneel by your partner's side. Place your hands over each side of his midriff with your fingers pointing away. Glide your hands diagonally across each other to circle in opposite directions around both sides of his body.

2 ◁ Slide your hands back past each other to encircle the opposite sides. Repeat the figure-of-eight action as required, varying the tempo, speed, and pressure to add variety and vitality. Take the stroke in a continuous, unbroken flowing action up and down the torso.

73 CROSS-OVERS

Slide your hands past each other across the belly in a smooth, unbroken action. Work up and down from the hips to the ribcage.

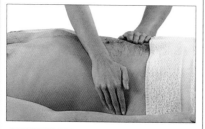

TAKE YOUR HANDS DOWN TO THE MATTRESS

74 MILKING STROKES

Pull one hand after the other over the side of the abdomen to create a milking action. Lift your hands when they reach the centre.

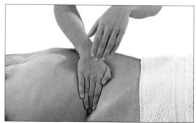

EMPHASIZE THE BODY'S SCULPTURED FORM

75 KNEAD THE WAIST

Kneel on the opposite side of the body to where you wish to knead. Hold your elbows away from your sides and knead and wring along the side of the abdomen where the muscles wrap around the body. Scoop, roll, and push the flesh with both hands up and down, from the pelvic girdle to the ribcage. Repeat on the other side of the body.

Keep your arms and hands supple

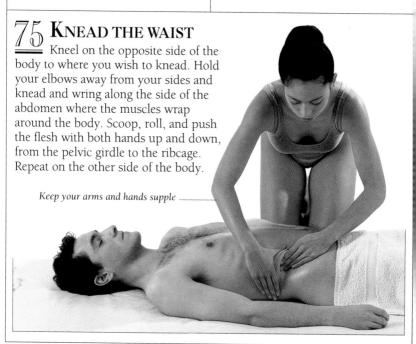

76 EASY BREATHING

The diaphragm is fundamental to the breathing process. It is too deep within the body to be reached by soft tissue massage, but relaxation of the area around the ribcage is helpful for breathing and relieves tension. Slip your right hand under the back and keep your left hand relaxed and raised slightly off the body. Sink the heel of this hand gently into the flesh and massage in circles below the ribcage.

HELP INHALATION
Massage around the diaphragm increases lung pressure.

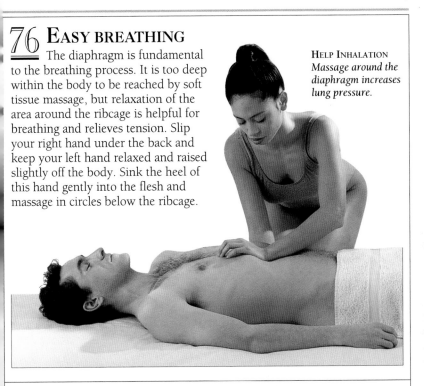

77 BELLY HOLD

Round off a belly massage with this cradling connection hold. Slip your right hand under the back to relax the belly area and lower back. Place your left hand gently on the abdomen. This brings warmth and encourages breathing, thereby drawing oxygen to the vital organs enclosed. Feel your partner's tension dissolve and his breathing deepen. Hold for a few minutes to achieve complete relaxation.

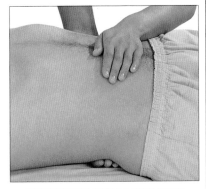

ALLOW TIME TO RESTORE EQUILIBRIUM

THE ARMS & HANDS

78 CONCENTRATE ON THE ARMS

A comprehensive massage of the hands and arms should include a range of strokes, including passive movements, effleurage, kneading, and petrissage. When all the strokes are completed, finish with delicate, feather-like touches down the arm using the fingertips of one hand, then the other. Repeat the complete sequence of strokes on the other arm.

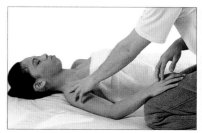

ARM STROKES BALANCE THE WHOLE BODY

79 LIFT AND STRETCH THE ARMS

Start off with passive movements to release tension from the joints and muscles of the arm. Take hold of your partner's hand in one hand and support the elbow with the other. Lift and lower the arm several times. When raised, give the arm a light pull to stretch the shoulder joint. Lower the arm and clasp the wrist with both hands. Lean back and pull to create a gentle arm stretch. Release the arm back into a relaxed position.

PROVIDE SUPPORT
Try to encourage your partner to let you take charge of the movement.

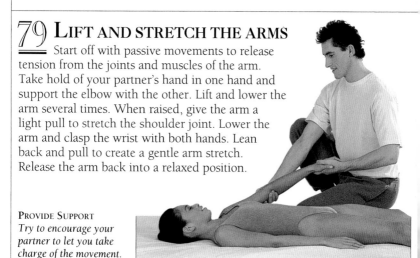

80 FLEX THE WRISTS

Use this stroke to increase mobility in wrists that have become stiff as a result of repetitive movements. Take hold of your partner's arm just above the wrist and hold onto the hand. Extend and flex the wrist by gently bending the hand back and forth. Conclude by rotating the hand gently left and right around the joint.

Never push the wrist beyond the extent of its natural motion

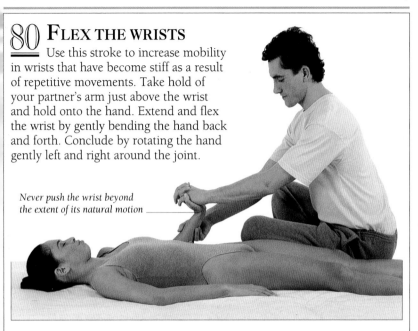

81 STROKING

Take one of your partner's hands in yours. Slide your other hand firmly up the arm and glide up and over the shoulder. Embrace the shoulder with both hands, one below and one above, and pull down the length of the arm. Pull in a firm stretch towards your body. Glide the stroke out of the hands and the end of the fingers.

82 KNEADING

Apply kneading strokes to ease tension in the arm muscles. Cup the arm with one hand, supporting it with the fingers. Work both thumbs along the muscles of the arm in alternate circular motions. Apply added pressure around the outward half-circle of the stroke and squeeze the flesh with your heels and thumbs.

83 PETRISSAGE

Take hold of your partner's hand in yours and raise her forearm a little distance from the mattress. Glide your thumb pad slowly but firmly up between the two long bones of the forearm, the radius and the ulna. Take the action up as far as the elbow joint. Follow up with effleurage strokes to the lower arm.

THE ARMS & HANDS

84 HAND MASSAGE

Give a hand massage before or after an arm massage for added relaxation and suppleness. A hand massage is simple and quick to give, requires minimum preparation, and can take place anywhere. Hands are hard-working parts of the body, so it is deeply comforting for them to be pampered for a change. Massage one hand at a time, keeping your wrists relaxed. Repeat the sequence of strokes on the other hand.

- Begin with a simple hand-hold to comfort and reassure your partner.
- Support the hand as you work.
- Massage to stimulate the nerve endings in the fingertips and palms.

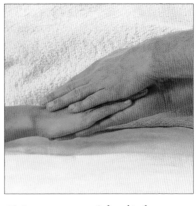

1 Lay your partner's hand in between yours and hold it gently for a few moments. This is a very calming action. The warmth of your hands will release tension and give a feeling of tranquillity.

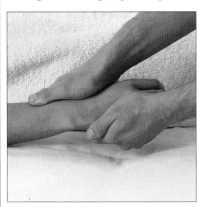

2 Manipulate the bones and tendons of the hand to make it more supple. Supporting the palm with your fingers, make circular motions with your heels and thumbs, from the base of the fingers to the wrist, one hand after the other.

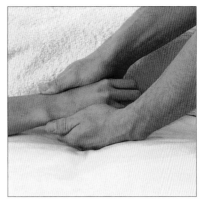

3 Remove tension from your partner's hand with a stretching stroke. Slide your thumbs and the heels of your hands from the centre to the sides of the hand. Support the palm with your fingers as you stretch across the upper hand.

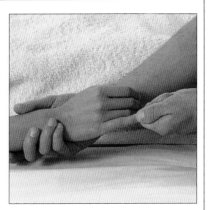

4 Support your partner's hand with the palm facing downwards. Use your thumb and index finger to pull along the length of each finger, right down to the tip. Squeeze the end of each finger.

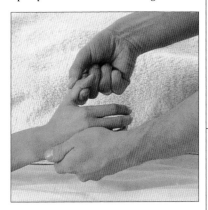

5 Take hold of your partner's thumb between the thumb and forefinger. Pull and squeeze as you did with the fingers. Massage the base, using your heel and fingertips. Press into the web of flesh between thumb and forefinger.

85 RELAX STIFFNESS

Use this stroke to increase flexibility in the hand by reducing stiffness in the ligaments of the wrist. Support your partner's hand or forearm on your thigh or in your hand. Her elbow should remain flexed to avoid straining the joint with the weight of her arm. Make small, alternate, circular movements of the thumbs over the palm of the hand, moving gradually up to stroke the soft skin around the wrist.

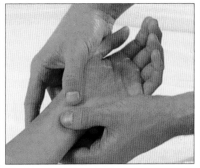

USE ONLY GENTLE PRESSURE ON THE WRIST

86 HAND ANATOMY

There are 27 bones in each hand, which are mobilized by muscles attached to the bones in the upper arm and forearm. Tendons create movement in the palm and fingers. Thousands of nerve endings in the fingers and palm increase the satisfying and stimulating effect of a hand massage on the whole body.

THE LEGS & FEET

87 CRADLE THE FOOT

Position yourself at your partner's feet. Use cushions if necessary to support your own posture. Start off a foot massage by cradling the foot between your hands. Focus on your breathing and concentrate on the soothing quality of your touch. This initial simple action will calm the whole person by drawing attention away from a busy, over-stimulated mind, down the body, to produce a highly restful effect.

WHOLE-BODY BENEFITS
The soles of the feet hold thousands of nerve endings. Use foot massage to stimulate the physiological system and to ease postural tension in the feet and legs.

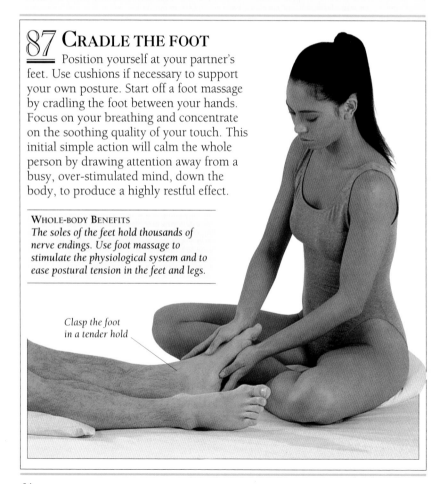

Clasp the foot in a tender hold

88 STROKE THE FOOT

Place both hands parallel on the foot, little fingers leading. Glide your hands down from the toes to the ankles. Draw your hands out around both sides of the ankle bone and stroke your fingers along the sole. Repeat the action several times.

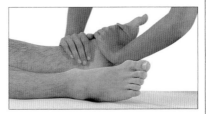

LET THE LITTLE FINGERS LEAD THE STROKE

89 SPREAD THE FOOT

Hook your fingers around the sole of the foot and slide your heels and thumbs out to both edges of the instep. Work the stroke up towards the ankle. This outward stretch will create a pleasant feeling of width and space in the foot.

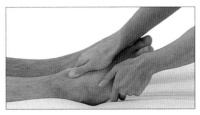

CREATE A SATISFYING STRETCH

90 WORK THE SOLE

Use the broad surface of the heel of the hand to make circular strokes along the sole, up the sides of the foot and arches, and over the instep. This will help to improve the entire body posture and revitalize the supply of blood to the foot.

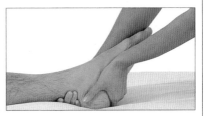

PRESSURE ON THE SOLES DISPELS TOXINS

91 WORK THE ANKLE

Raise the foot with one hand and stroke around the outer ankle bone with the fingertips of the other. Apply gentle petrissage in small circles near the bone, one area at a time. Manipulate the tissue in the same way on the inner bone.

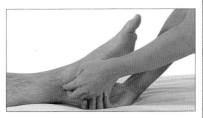

ALWAYS KEEP THE ANKLE FLEXIBLE

92 STROKE BETWEEN THE TENDONS

Raise and support the foot with one hand and use the heel of one hand and then the other to rub both sides of the Achilles tendon. Gently lower the foot to the mattress and move your hands round to work on the tendons on the instep. Slide your thumbs along the grooves between each tendon, from the base of the toes along the length of the instep up to the ankle.

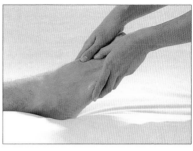

RELAX THE TENDONS OF THE UPPER FOOT

93 MASSAGE FOR TOES

The toes store a surprising amount of tension, which is why passive movement and massage of each toe has such a beneficial effect on the whole body. Support your partner's foot with one hand and use the other hand to work along from the big toe to the little toe. Change hands as necessary.

- Poor posture may sometimes result in tension in the toes. This is because the body weight is not evenly distributed across the feet.
- The soft skin that lies in between the big toe and the second toe is particularly sensitive to touch, so be careful not to tickle your partner.
- Don't pull the toes too hard.

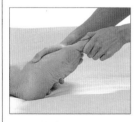

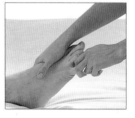

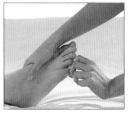

1 Hold the upper foot and grasp the big toe between the thumb and forefinger. Pull along the toe steadily from base to top and squeeze the tip.

2 Stroke along the sides of the toe by clasping the base between your forefinger and middle finger and pulling the toe towards your body.

3 Hold the end of the toe between your fingertips and wiggle the joints up and down. Rotate the toe and squeeze gently along its length.

94 SHIN SLIDE

Begin by oiling the leg and relaxing it with long, flowing strokes followed by fan strokes. To release tension from the lower leg, apply a deep petrissage stroke between the shin bones. Sink your thumb pad into the groove between the two long bones and glide it smoothly from the ankle to the knee.

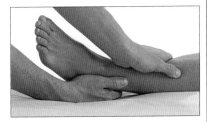

REPEAT THREE TIMES TO RELIEVE STRAIN

95 RELAX THE KNEES

Slip your fingers underneath the knee for support and use your thumb pads to glide around the circumference of the kneecap, from the top to the base and back up again. Repeat several times. Then make small rotations above the kneecap with your thumb pads. Apply firm but gentle pressure.

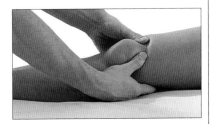

RELAX THE LIGAMENTS TO AID MOBILITY

96 LONG LEG STRETCH

Warm the thigh with fan strokes, circle strokes, then kneading. Continue with several main effleurage strokes that glide from foot to thigh before sliding back down each side of the leg and drawing out of the foot. Repeat all strokes on the other leg.

Adjust your position as you move up and down each leg

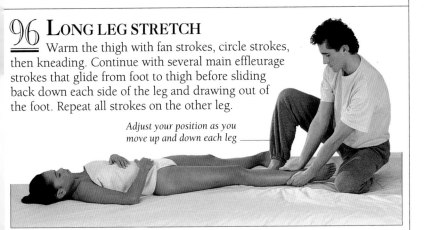

THE FINISH

97 HOW TO CONCLUDE

A good massage deserves a fitting conclusion. Try to make as much effort with the closing stages as with the rest of the massage sequence to leave your partner feeling comfortable and relaxed. After becoming accustomed to your touch, he may feel abandoned if you end the session too abruptly.

98 FINAL HOLD

Choose any part of the body for a final energy balancing hold. The soles of the feet or crown of the head are best for achieving a sense of balance and bringing about a feeling of rest. Keep your hands in place and focus your attention on your partner for at least a minute. Withdraw your hands slowly.

99 ENJOY THE EFFECTS

Your partner will need time to assimilate the effects of the massage. He should feel relaxed and peaceful, but he may also feel vulnerable after the gradual release of physical and emotional tension. He will need time to lie back and absorb the effects.

KEEP IN TOUCH
Maintain contact with your partner's hand while he relaxes.

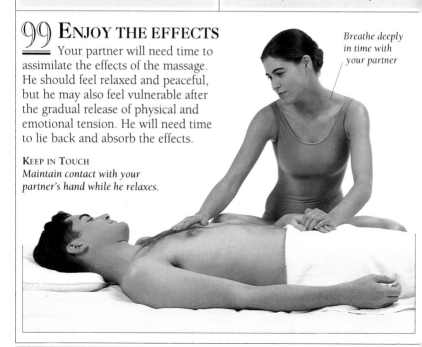

Breathe deeply in time with your partner

100 THE REST POSITION

Your partner may wish to relax a while longer at the end of the session. Ask him to turn over and rest on his side. It can be comforting to feel the actual physical presence of someone close – if appropriate you can lie alongside. Place your hand on his body for reassurance.

KEEP COMFORTABLE
Don't put any strain on your own posture as you lie beside your partner. He will sense that you are not relaxed.

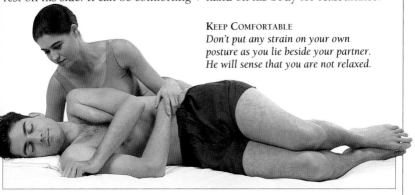

101 GETTING UP

When your partner is ready to get up, be there to help him to sit upright and to lever himself up without putting strain on his back. It is common for recipients to feel so relaxed at the end of a massage that they are disorientated and need support for a few moments in order to feel totally stable.

MUTUAL APPRECIATION
Take this opportunity to thank each other for the pleasure of giving and receiving a massage.

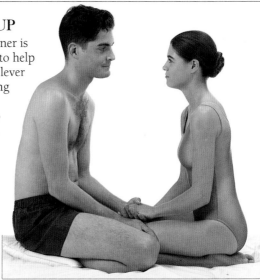

INDEX

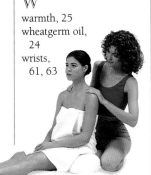

Acknowledgments

Dorling Kindersley would like to thank Hilary Bird for compiling the index; Ann Kay for proof-reading; Bella Pringle for editorial assistance; Murdo Culver for design assistance; Mark Bracey for computer assistance; Paula Atkinson, Isabelle Hassé, Jonathan Stigwood, Daniel Talone, and Rokiah Yaman for modelling; Bettina Graham for hair and make-up; Rebecca Davies and Steve Pople for the loan of props.

Photography
All photographs by Jo Foord and Tim Ridley except for:
Antonia Deutsch 20, 21.

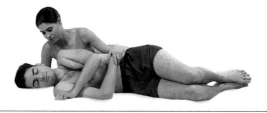